Caregiver Log Bo

This Book Belongs To:

Name: ....

Email: ....

Address: ....

Phone: ....

Care Recipient Info:

Name: ....

Email: ....

Address: ....

Phone: ....

Emergency Contacts:

Name: ....

Email: ....

Address: ....

Phone: ....

Name: ....

Email: ....

Address: ....

Phone: ....

Medical Health History

Medical Health History

Medical Health History

Caregiver Log Book

DATE ___ / ___ / ___   MON TUE WED THU FRI SAT SUN

Patient Name: ....

Caregiver: ....

Weight	Blood Pressure	Feeling

Food Consumption	Time

Medication	Dosage	Time

Activities

....

....

....

Caregiver Log Book

DATE _____ / _____ / _____   MON   TUE   WED   THU   FRI   SAT   SUN

Patient Name: ....

Caregiver: ....

Weight	Blood Pressure	Feeling

Food Consumption	Time

Medication	Dosage	Time

Activities ....

....

....

....

Caregiver Log Book

DATE _____ / _____ / _____   MON   TUE   WED   THU   FRI   SAT   SUN

Patient Name: ....

Caregiver: ....

Weight	Blood Pressure	Feeling

Food Consumption	Time

Medication	Dosage	Time

Activities
....
....
....
....

Caregiver Log Book

DATE _____ / ___ / _____   MON TUE WED THU FRI SAT SUN

Patient Name: ....

Caregiver: ....

Weight	Blood Pressure	Feeling

Food Consumption	Time

Medication	Dosage	Time

Activities

....

....

....

Caregiver Log Book

DATE _____ / _____ / _____   MON   TUE   WED   THU   FRI   SAT   SUN

Patient Name: ....

Caregiver: ....

Weight	Blood Pressure	Feeling

Food Consumption	Time

Medication	Dosage	Time

Activities

....

....

....

....

Caregiver Log Book

DATE _____ / _____ / _____   MON   TUE   WED   THU   FRI   SAT   SUN

Patient Name: ....

Caregiver: ....

Weight	Blood Pressure	Feeling

Food Consumption	Time

Medication	Dosage	Time

Activities

....

....

....

Caregiver Log Book

DATE ___ / ___ / ___   MON TUE WED THU FRI SAT SUN

Patient Name: ....

Caregiver: ....

Weight	Blood Pressure	Feeling

Food Consumption	Time

Medication	Dosage	Time

Activities ....

....

....

....

Caregiver Log Book

DATE ___ / ___ / ___   MON TUE WED THU FRI SAT SUN

Patient Name: ....

Caregiver: ....

Weight	Blood Pressure	Feeling

Food Consumption	Time

Medication	Dosage	Time

Activities

....

....

....

Caregiver Log Book

DATE ___ / ___ / ___   MON TUE WED THU FRI SAT SUN

Patient Name: ....

Caregiver: ....

Weight	Blood Pressure	Feeling

Food Consumption	Time

Medication	Dosage	Time

Activities

....

....

....

Caregiver Log Book

DATE ___/___/___   MON   TUE   WED   THU   FRI   SAT   SUN

Patient Name: ....

Caregiver: ....

Weight	Blood Pressure	Feeling

Food Consumption	Time

Medication	Dosage	Time

Activities

....

....

....

Caregiver Log Book

DATE _____ / ___ / _____   MON TUE WED THU FRI SAT SUN

Patient Name: ....

Caregiver: ....

Weight	Blood Pressure	Feeling

Food Consumption	Time

Medication	Dosage	Time

Activities ....

....

....

....

Caregiver Log Book

DATE ____/____/____   MON TUE WED THU FRI SAT SUN

Patient Name: ....

Caregiver: ....

Weight	Blood Pressure	Feeling

Food Consumption	Time

Medication	Dosage	Time

Activities

....

....

....

Caregiver Log Book

DATE ___ / ___ / ___   MON TUE WED THU FRI SAT SUN

Patient Name: ....

Caregiver: ....

Weight	Blood Pressure	Feeling

Food Consumption	Time

Medication	Dosage	Time

Activities

....

....

....

Caregiver Log Book

DATE ___/___/___   MON TUE WED THU FRI SAT SUN

Patient Name: ....

Caregiver: ....

Weight	Blood Pressure	Feeling

Food Consumption	Time

Medication	Dosage	Time

Activities ....

....

....

....

Caregiver Log Book

DATE _____ / ___ / _____   MON TUE WED THU FRI SAT SUN

Patient Name: ....

Caregiver: ....

Weight	Blood Pressure	Feeling

Food Consumption	Time

Medication	Dosage	Time

Activities
....
....
....

Caregiver Log Book

DATE ___ / ___ / ___   MON TUE WED THU FRI SAT SUN

Patient Name: ....

Caregiver: ....

Weight	Blood Pressure	Feeling

Food Consumption	Time

Medication	Dosage	Time

Activities

....

....

....

....

Caregiver Log Book

DATE _____ / _____ / _____   MON TUE WED THU FRI SAT SUN

Patient Name: ....

Caregiver: ....

Weight	Blood Pressure	Feeling

Food Consumption	Time

Medication	Dosage	Time

Activities
....

....

....

....

Caregiver Log Book

DATE ____/____/____   MON TUE WED THU FRI SAT SUN

Patient Name: ....

Caregiver: ....

Weight	Blood Pressure	Feeling

Food Consumption	Time

Medication	Dosage	Time

Activities

....

....

....

Caregiver Log Book

DATE ____ / ____ / ____   MON TUE WED THU FRI SAT SUN

Patient Name: ....

Caregiver: ....

Weight	Blood Pressure	Feeling

Food Consumption	Time

Medication	Dosage	Time

Activities ....

....

....

....

Caregiver Log Book

DATE ___/___/___   MON TUE WED THU FRI SAT SUN

Patient Name: ....

Caregiver: ....

Weight	Blood Pressure	Feeling

Food Consumption	Time

Medication	Dosage	Time

Activities

....

....

....

Caregiver Log Book

DATE ___ / ___ / ___   MON TUE WED THU FRI SAT SUN

Patient Name: ....

Caregiver: ....

Weight	Blood Pressure	Feeling

Food Consumption	Time

Medication	Dosage	Time

Activities
....

....

....

Caregiver Log Book

DATE ___/___/___   MON   TUE   WED   THU   FRI   SAT   SUN

Patient Name: ....

Caregiver: ....

Weight	Blood Pressure	Feeling

Food Consumption	Time

Medication	Dosage	Time

Activities

....

....

....

....

Caregiver Log Book

DATE ___/___/___ MON TUE WED THU FRI SAT SUN

Patient Name: ....

Caregiver: ....

Weight	Blood Pressure	Feeling

Food Consumption	Time

Medication	Dosage	Time

Activities

....

....

....

Caregiver Log Book

DATE _____/_____/_____   MON   TUE   WED   THU   FRI   SAT   SUN

Patient Name: ....

Caregiver: ....

Weight	Blood Pressure	Feeling

Food Consumption	Time

Medication	Dosage	Time

Activities

....

....

....

Caregiver Log Book

DATE _____ / _____ / _____   MON TUE WED THU FRI SAT SUN

Patient Name: ....

Caregiver: ....

Weight	Blood Pressure	Feeling

Food Consumption	Time

Medication	Dosage	Time

Activities ....

....

....

....

Caregiver Log Book

DATE ___ / ___ / ___   MON   TUE   WED   THU   FRI   SAT   SUN

Patient Name: ....

Caregiver: ....

Weight	Blood Pressure	Feeling

Food Consumption	Time

Medication	Dosage	Time

Activities ....

....

....

....

Caregiver Log Book

DATE ____ / ____ / ____   MON   TUE   WED   THU   FRI   SAT   SUN

Patient Name: ....

Caregiver: ....

Weight	Blood Pressure	Feeling

Food Consumption	Time

Medication	Dosage	Time

Activities

....

....

....

....

Caregiver Log Book

DATE ____/____/____   MON   TUE   WED   THU   FRI   SAT   SUN

Patient Name: ....

Caregiver: ....

Weight	Blood Pressure	Feeling

Food Consumption	Time

Medication	Dosage	Time

Activities

....

....

....

Caregiver Log Book

DATE ____/____/____ MON TUE WED THU FRI SAT SUN

Patient Name: ....

Caregiver: ....

Weight	Blood Pressure	Feeling

Food Consumption	Time

Medication	Dosage	Time

Activities
....
....
....

Caregiver Log Book

DATE ___/___/___   MON TUE WED THU FRI SAT SUN

Patient Name: ....

Caregiver: ....

Weight	Blood Pressure	Feeling

Food Consumption	Time

Medication	Dosage	Time

Activities

....

....

....

....

Caregiver Log Book

DATE _____ / _____ / _____   MON   TUE   WED   THU   FRI   SAT   SUN

Patient Name: ....

Caregiver: ....

Weight	Blood Pressure	Feeling

Food Consumption	Time

Medication	Dosage	Time

Activities

....

....

....

Caregiver Log Book

DATE ____/____/____   MON TUE WED THU FRI SAT SUN

Patient Name: ....

Caregiver: ....

Weight	Blood Pressure	Feeling

Food Consumption	Time

Medication	Dosage	Time

Activities

....

....

....

Caregiver Log Book

DATE _____/_____/_____   MON TUE WED THU FRI SAT SUN

Patient Name: ....

Caregiver: ....

Weight	Blood Pressure	Feeling

Food Consumption

Food Consumption	Time

Medication	Dosage	Time

Activities

....

....

....

....

Caregiver Log Book

DATE ___/___/___   MON TUE WED THU FRI SAT SUN

Patient Name: ....

Caregiver: ....

Weight	Blood Pressure	Feeling

Food Consumption	Time

Medication	Dosage	Time

Activities ....

....

....

....

Caregiver Log Book

DATE ___ / ___ / ___   MON TUE WED THU FRI SAT SUN

Patient Name: ....

Caregiver: ....

Weight	Blood Pressure	Feeling

Food Consumption	Time

Medication	Dosage	Time

Activities

....

....

....

....

Caregiver Log Book

DATE ___ / ___ / ___   MON   TUE   WED   THU   FRI   SAT   SUN

Patient Name: ....

Caregiver: ....

Weight	Blood Pressure	Feeling

Food Consumption	Time

Medication	Dosage	Time

Activities

....

....

....

Caregiver Log Book

DATE _____ / _____ / _____   MON   TUE   WED   THU   FRI   SAT   SUN

Patient Name: ....

Caregiver: ....

Weight	Blood Pressure	Feeling

Food Consumption	Time

Medication	Dosage	Time

Activities
....

....

....

Caregiver Log Book

DATE _____ / _____ / _____   MON   TUE   WED   THU   FRI   SAT   SUN

Patient Name: ....

Caregiver: ....

Weight	Blood Pressure	Feeling

Food Consumption	Time

Medication	Dosage	Time

Activities
....
....
....
....

Caregiver Log Book

DATE _____ / _____ / _____   MON   TUE   WED   THU   FRI   SAT   SUN

Patient Name: ....

Caregiver: ....

Weight	Blood Pressure	Feeling

Food Consumption	Time

Medication	Dosage	Time

Activities ....

....

....

....

Caregiver Log Book

DATE _____ / _____ / _____   MON TUE WED THU FRI SAT SUN

Patient Name: ....

Caregiver: ....

Weight	Blood Pressure	Feeling

Food Consumption	Time

Medication	Dosage	Time

Activities
....

....

....

....

Caregiver Log Book

DATE ____ / ____ / ____   MON TUE WED THU FRI SAT SUN

Patient Name: ....

Caregiver: ....

Weight	Blood Pressure	Feeling

Food Consumption	Time

Medication	Dosage	Time

Activities

....

....

....

Caregiver Log Book

DATE ____ / ____ / ____   MON   TUE   WED   THU   FRI   SAT   SUN

Patient Name: ....

Caregiver: ....

Weight	Blood Pressure	Feeling

Food Consumption	Time

Medication	Dosage	Time

Activities ....

....

....

....

Caregiver Log Book

DATE ___ / ___ / ___   MON TUE WED THU FRI SAT SUN

Patient Name: ....

Caregiver: ....

Weight	Blood Pressure	Feeling

Food Consumption	Time

Medication	Dosage	Time

Activities

....

....

....

Caregiver Log Book

DATE _____ / ___ / _____   MON   TUE   WED   THU   FRI   SAT   SUN

Patient Name: ....

Caregiver: ....

Weight	Blood Pressure	Feeling

Food Consumption	Time

Medication	Dosage	Time

Activities

....

....

....

Caregiver Log Book

DATE _____ / _____ / _____   MON TUE WED THU FRI SAT SUN

Patient Name: ....

Caregiver: ....

Weight	Blood Pressure	Feeling

Food Consumption	Time

Medication	Dosage	Time

Activities
....

....

....

Caregiver Log Book

DATE ___/___/___ MON TUE WED THU FRI SAT SUN

Patient Name: ....

Caregiver: ....

Weight	Blood Pressure	Feeling

Food Consumption	Time

Medication	Dosage	Time

Activities

....

....

....

Caregiver Log Book

DATE ___ / ___ / ___   MON TUE WED THU FRI SAT SUN

Patient Name: ....

Caregiver: ....

Weight	Blood Pressure	Feeling

Food Consumption	Time

Medication	Dosage	Time

Activities

....

....

....

Caregiver Log Book

DATE ___/___/___   MON TUE WED THU FRI SAT SUN

Patient Name: ....

Caregiver: ....

Weight	Blood Pressure	Feeling

Food Consumption	Time

Medication	Dosage	Time

Activities

....

....

....

Caregiver Log Book

DATE _____ / _____ / _____ MON TUE WED THU FRI SAT SUN

Patient Name: ....

Caregiver: ....

Weight	Blood Pressure	Feeling

Food Consumption	Time

Medication	Dosage	Time

Activities ....

....

....

....

Caregiver Log Book

DATE _____ / ___ / _____   MON TUE WED THU FRI SAT SUN

Patient Name: ....

Caregiver: ....

Weight	Blood Pressure	Feeling

Food Consumption	Time

Medication	Dosage	Time

Activities

....

....

....

Caregiver Log Book

DATE ___ / ___ / ___   MON TUE WED THU FRI SAT SUN

Patient Name: ....

Caregiver: ....

Weight	Blood Pressure	Feeling

Food Consumption	Time

Medication	Dosage	Time

Activities
....
....
....

Caregiver Log Book

DATE ____ / ____ / ____   MON TUE WED THU FRI SAT SUN

Patient Name: ....

Caregiver: ....

Weight	Blood Pressure	Feeling

Food Consumption	Time

Medication	Dosage	Time

Activities

....

....

....

Caregiver Log Book

DATE _____ / _____ / _____   MON TUE WED THU FRI SAT SUN

Patient Name: ....

Caregiver: ....

Weight	Blood Pressure	Feeling

Food Consumption	Time

Medication	Dosage	Time

Activities
....

....

....

....

Caregiver Log Book

DATE _____ / _____ / _____   MON TUE WED THU FRI SAT SUN

Patient Name: ....

Caregiver: ....

Weight	Blood Pressure	Feeling

Food Consumption	Time

Medication	Dosage	Time

Activities

....

....

....

Caregiver Log Book

DATE ____ / ____ / ____   MON TUE WED THU FRI SAT SUN

Patient Name: ....

Caregiver: ....

Weight	Blood Pressure	Feeling

Food Consumption	Time

Medication	Dosage	Time

Activities ....

....

....

....

Caregiver Log Book

DATE ___ / ___ / ___   MON   TUE   WED   THU   FRI   SAT   SUN

Patient Name: ....

Caregiver: ....

Weight	Blood Pressure	Feeling

Food Consumption	Time

Medication	Dosage	Time

Activities

....

....

....

....

Caregiver Log Book

DATE ___ / ___ / ___   MON TUE WED THU FRI SAT SUN

Patient Name: ....

Caregiver: ....

Weight	Blood Pressure	Feeling

Food Consumption	Time

Medication	Dosage	Time

Activities
....

....

....

Caregiver Log Book

DATE ____ / ____ / ____   MON   TUE   WED   THU   FRI   SAT   SUN

Patient Name: ....

Caregiver: ....

Weight	Blood Pressure	Feeling

Food Consumption	Time

Medication	Dosage	Time

Activities

....

....

....

Caregiver Log Book

DATE ___/___/___   MON TUE WED THU FRI SAT SUN

Patient Name: ....

Caregiver: ....

Weight	Blood Pressure	Feeling

Food Consumption	Time

Medication	Dosage	Time

Activities

....

....

....

Caregiver Log Book

DATE ___/___/___ MON TUE WED THU FRI SAT SUN

Patient Name: ....

Caregiver: ....

Weight	Blood Pressure	Feeling

Food Consumption	Time

Medication	Dosage	Time

Activities

....

....

....

Caregiver Log Book

DATE ___ / ___ / ___   MON TUE WED THU FRI SAT SUN

Patient Name: ....

Caregiver: ....

Weight	Blood Pressure	Feeling

Food Consumption	Time

Medication	Dosage	Time

Activities ....

....

....

....

Caregiver Log Book

DATE _____/___/_____   MON   TUE   WED   THU   FRI   SAT   SUN

Patient Name: ....

Caregiver: ....

Weight	Blood Pressure	Feeling

Food Consumption	Time

Medication	Dosage	Time

Activities

....

....

....

Caregiver Log Book

DATE _____ / _____ / _____   MON TUE WED THU FRI SAT SUN

Patient Name: ....

Caregiver: ....

Weight	Blood Pressure	Feeling

Food Consumption	Time

Medication	Dosage	Time

Activities

....

....

....

Caregiver Log Book

DATE ____/____/____   MON TUE WED THU FRI SAT SUN

Patient Name: ....

Caregiver: ....

Weight	Blood Pressure	Feeling

Food Consumption	Time

Medication	Dosage	Time

Activities

....

....

....

Caregiver Log Book

DATE ___ / ___ / ___   MON   TUE   WED   THU   FRI   SAT   SUN

Patient Name: ....

Caregiver: ....

Weight	Blood Pressure	Feeling

Food Consumption	Time

Medication	Dosage	Time

Activities
....
....
....
....

Caregiver Log Book

DATE ____/____/____ MON TUE WED THU FRI SAT SUN

Patient Name: ....

Caregiver: ....

Weight	Blood Pressure	Feeling

Food Consumption	Time

Medication	Dosage	Time

Activities

....

....

....

Caregiver Log Book

DATE _____/_____/_____ MON TUE WED THU FRI SAT SUN

Patient Name: ....

Caregiver: ....

Weight	Blood Pressure	Feeling

Food Consumption	Time

Medication	Dosage	Time

Activities

....

....

....

....

Caregiver Log Book

DATE ____/____/____   MON TUE WED THU FRI SAT SUN

Patient Name: ....

Caregiver: ....

Weight	Blood Pressure	Feeling

Food Consumption	Time

Medication	Dosage	Time

Activities
....
....
....

Caregiver Log Book

DATE ___/___/___ MON TUE WED THU FRI SAT SUN

Patient Name: ....

Caregiver: ....

Weight	Blood Pressure	Feeling

Food Consumption	Time

Medication	Dosage	Time

Activities ....

....

....

....

Caregiver Log Book

DATE ___/___/___   MON TUE WED THU FRI SAT SUN

Patient Name: ....

Caregiver: ....

Weight	Blood Pressure	Feeling

Food Consumption	Time

Medication	Dosage	Time

Activities

....

....

....

Caregiver Log Book

DATE ___ / ___ / ___   MON TUE WED THU FRI SAT SUN

Patient Name: ....

Caregiver: ....

Weight	Blood Pressure	Feeling

Food Consumption	Time

Medication	Dosage	Time

Activities

....

....

....

Caregiver Log Book

DATE _____ / ___ / _____   MON TUE WED THU FRI SAT SUN

Patient Name: ....

Caregiver: ....

Weight	Blood Pressure	Feeling

Food Consumption	Time

Medication	Dosage	Time

Activities

....

....

....

Caregiver Log Book

DATE ___/___/___   MON TUE WED THU FRI SAT SUN

Patient Name: ....

Caregiver: ....

Weight	Blood Pressure	Feeling

Food Consumption	Time

Medication	Dosage	Time

Activities
....

....

....

Caregiver Log Book

DATE ___ / ___ / ___   MON TUE WED THU FRI SAT SUN

Patient Name: ....

Caregiver: ....

Weight	Blood Pressure	Feeling

Food Consumption	Time

Medication	Dosage	Time

Activities

....

....

....

....

Caregiver Log Book

DATE _____ / _____ / _____   MON TUE WED THU FRI SAT SUN

Patient Name: ....

Caregiver: ....

Weight	Blood Pressure	Feeling

Food Consumption	Time

Medication	Dosage	Time

Activities ....

....

....

....

Caregiver Log Book

DATE _____ / _____ / _____   MON TUE WED THU FRI SAT SUN

Patient Name: ....

Caregiver: ....

Weight	Blood Pressure	Feeling

Food Consumption	Time

Medication	Dosage	Time

Activities
....
....
....

Caregiver Log Book

DATE _____/_____/_____   MON   TUE   WED   THU   FRI   SAT   SUN

Patient Name: ....

Caregiver: ....

Weight	Blood Pressure	Feeling

Food Consumption	Time

Medication	Dosage	Time

Activities
....

....

....

Caregiver Log Book

DATE ___/___/___   MON   TUE   WED   THU   FRI   SAT   SUN

Patient Name: ....

Caregiver: ....

Weight	Blood Pressure	Feeling

Food Consumption	Time

Medication	Dosage	Time

Activities

....

....

....

....

Caregiver Log Book

DATE ___/___/___ MON TUE WED THU FRI SAT SUN

Patient Name: ....

Caregiver: ....

Weight	Blood Pressure	Feeling

Food Consumption	Time

Medication	Dosage	Time

Activities ....

....

....

....

Caregiver Log Book

DATE _____/_____/_____   MON   TUE   WED   THU   FRI   SAT   SUN

Patient Name: ....

Caregiver: ....

Weight	Blood Pressure	Feeling

Food Consumption	Time

Medication	Dosage	Time

Activities

....

....

....

Caregiver Log Book

DATE _____/___/_____   MON TUE WED THU FRI SAT SUN

Patient Name: ....

Caregiver: ....

Weight	Blood Pressure	Feeling

Food Consumption	Time

Medication	Dosage	Time

Activities ....

....

....

....

Caregiver Log Book

DATE _____ / _____ / _____   MON TUE WED THU FRI SAT SUN

Patient Name: ....

Caregiver: ....

Weight	Blood Pressure	Feeling

Food Consumption	Time

Medication	Dosage	Time

Activities
....
....
....

Caregiver Log Book

DATE _____ / ___ / _____   MON TUE WED THU FRI SAT SUN

Patient Name: ....

Caregiver: ....

Weight	Blood Pressure	Feeling

Food Consumption	Time

Medication	Dosage	Time

Activities
....

....

....

....

Caregiver Log Book

DATE _____/_____/_____   MON TUE WED THU FRI SAT SUN

Patient Name: ....

Caregiver: ....

Weight	Blood Pressure	Feeling

Food Consumption	Time

Medication	Dosage	Time

Activities
....
....
....
....

Caregiver Log Book

DATE ____ / ____ / ____   MON TUE WED THU FRI SAT SUN

Patient Name: ....

Caregiver: ....

Weight	Blood Pressure	Feeling

Food Consumption

Food Consumption	Time

Medication

Medication	Dosage	Time

Activities

....

....

....

....

Caregiver Log Book

DATE _____ / ___ / _____   MON TUE WED THU FRI SAT SUN

Patient Name: ....

Caregiver: ....

Weight	Blood Pressure	Feeling

Food Consumption	Time

Medication	Dosage	Time

Activities

....

....

....

Caregiver Log Book

DATE _____ / _____ / _____   MON TUE WED THU FRI SAT SUN

Patient Name: ....

Caregiver: ....

Weight	Blood Pressure	Feeling

Food Consumption	Time

Medication	Dosage	Time

Activities ....

....

....

....

Caregiver Log Book

DATE ___ / ___ / ___   MON   TUE   WED   THU   FRI   SAT   SUN

Patient Name: ....

Caregiver: ....

Weight	Blood Pressure	Feeling

Food Consumption	Time

Medication	Dosage	Time

Activities

....

....

....

Caregiver Log Book

DATE ___ / ___ / ___   MON   TUE   WED   THU   FRI   SAT   SUN

Patient Name: ....

Caregiver: ....

Weight	Blood Pressure	Feeling

Food Consumption	Time

Medication	Dosage	Time

Activities
....

....

....

Caregiver Log Book

DATE _____ / ____ / _____   MON   TUE   WED   THU   FRI   SAT   SUN

Patient Name: ....

Caregiver: ....

Weight	Blood Pressure	Feeling

Food Consumption	Time

Medication	Dosage	Time

Activities
....

....

....

Caregiver Log Book

DATE ___ / ___ / ___   MON TUE WED THU FRI SAT SUN

Patient Name: ....

Caregiver: ....

Weight	Blood Pressure	Feeling

Food Consumption	Time

Medication	Dosage	Time

Activities

....

....

....

Caregiver Log Book

DATE _____ / ___ / _____   MON TUE WED THU FRI SAT SUN

Patient Name: ....

Caregiver: ....

Weight	Blood Pressure	Feeling

Food Consumption	Time

Medication	Dosage	Time

Activities

....

....

....

Caregiver Log Book

DATE ___ / ___ / ___   MON TUE WED THU FRI SAT SUN

Patient Name: ....

Caregiver: ....

Weight	Blood Pressure	Feeling

Food Consumption

Food Consumption	Time

Medication	Dosage	Time

Activities

....

....

....

Caregiver Log Book

DATE ___ / ___ / ___   MON TUE WED THU FRI SAT SUN

Patient Name: ....

Caregiver: ....

Weight	Blood Pressure	Feeling

Food Consumption	Time

Medication	Dosage	Time

Activities

....

....

....

Caregiver Log Book

DATE ____ / ____ / ____   MON TUE WED THU FRI SAT SUN

Patient Name: ....

Caregiver: ....

Weight	Blood Pressure	Feeling

Food Consumption	Time

Medication	Dosage	Time

Activities ....

....

....

....

Caregiver Log Book

DATE ____ / ____ / ____   MON TUE WED THU FRI SAT SUN

Patient Name: ....

Caregiver: ....

Weight	Blood Pressure	Feeling

Food Consumption	Time

Medication	Dosage	Time

Activities

....

....

....

Caregiver Log Book

DATE ___/___/___ MON TUE WED THU FRI SAT SUN

Patient Name: ....

Caregiver: ....

Weight	Blood Pressure	Feeling

Food Consumption	Time

Medication	Dosage	Time

Activities
....
....
....

Caregiver Log Book

DATE ____/____/____   MON TUE WED THU FRI SAT SUN

Patient Name: ....

Caregiver: ....

Weight	Blood Pressure	Feeling

Food Consumption	Time

Medication	Dosage	Time

Activities

....

....

....

....

Caregiver Log Book

DATE _____ / ___ / _____   MON   TUE   WED   THU   FRI   SAT   SUN

Patient Name: ....

Caregiver: ....

Weight	Blood Pressure	Feeling

Food Consumption	Time

Medication	Dosage	Time

Activities ....

....

....

....

Caregiver Log Book

DATE ____/____/____   MON TUE WED THU FRI SAT SUN

Patient Name: ....

Caregiver: ....

Weight	Blood Pressure	Feeling

Food Consumption	Time

Medication	Dosage	Time

Activities

....

....

....

Caregiver Log Book

DATE _____ / _____ / _____   MON   TUE   WED   THU   FRI   SAT   SUN

Patient Name: ....

Caregiver: ....

Weight	Blood Pressure	Feeling

Food Consumption	Time

Medication	Dosage	Time

Activities

....

....

....

....

Caregiver Log Book

DATE ___/___/___   MON   TUE   WED   THU   FRI   SAT   SUN

Patient Name: ....

Caregiver: ....

Weight	Blood Pressure	Feeling

Food Consumption		Time

Medication	Dosage	Time

Activities

....

....

....

....

Caregiver Log Book

DATE ___ / ___ / ___   MON TUE WED THU FRI SAT SUN

Patient Name: ....

Caregiver: ....

Weight	Blood Pressure	Feeling

Food Consumption	Time

Medication	Dosage	Time

Activities
....

....

....

Caregiver Log Book

DATE ___ / ___ / ___   MON TUE WED THU FRI SAT SUN

Patient Name: ....

Caregiver: ....

Weight	Blood Pressure	Feeling

Food Consumption	Time

Medication	Dosage	Time

Activities
....

....

....

Caregiver Log Book

DATE ___ / ___ / ___   MON TUE WED THU FRI SAT SUN

Patient Name: ....

Caregiver: ....

Weight	Blood Pressure	Feeling

Food Consumption	Time

Medication	Dosage	Time

Activities ....

....

....

....

Caregiver Log Book

DATE ___/___/___ MON TUE WED THU FRI SAT SUN

Patient Name: ....

Caregiver: ....

Weight	Blood Pressure	Feeling

Food Consumption	Time

Medication	Dosage	Time

Activities

....

....

....

Caregiver Log Book

DATE _____ / _____ / _____   MON TUE WED THU FRI SAT SUN

Patient Name: ....

Caregiver: ....

Weight	Blood Pressure	Feeling

Food Consumption	Time

Medication	Dosage	Time

Activities

....

....

....

....

Caregiver Log Book

DATE _____ / ___ / _____   MON   TUE   WED   THU   FRI   SAT   SUN

Patient Name: ....

Caregiver: ....

Weight	Blood Pressure	Feeling

Food Consumption	Time

Medication	Dosage	Time

Activities

....

....

....

Caregiver Log Book

DATE ___ / ___ / ___   MON   TUE   WED   THU   FRI   SAT   SUN

Patient Name: ....

Caregiver: ....

Weight	Blood Pressure	Feeling

Food Consumption	Time

Medication	Dosage	Time

Activities
....

....

....

Caregiver Log Book

DATE ___/___/___   MON   TUE   WED   THU   FRI   SAT   SUN

Patient Name: ....

Caregiver: ....

Weight	Blood Pressure	Feeling

Food Consumption	Time

Medication	Dosage	Time

Activities

....

....

....

....

Caregiver Log Book

DATE ___ / ___ / ___   MON TUE WED THU FRI SAT SUN

Patient Name: ....

Caregiver: ....

Weight	Blood Pressure	Feeling

Food Consumption	Time

Medication	Dosage	Time

Activities ....

....

....

....

Caregiver Log Book

DATE ____/____/____   MON TUE WED THU FRI SAT SUN

Patient Name: ....

Caregiver: ....

Weight	Blood Pressure	Feeling

Food Consumption	Time

Medication	Dosage	Time

Activities

....

....

....

Caregiver Log Book

DATE ___/___/___   MON TUE WED THU FRI SAT SUN

Patient Name: ....

Caregiver: ....

Weight	Blood Pressure	Feeling

Food Consumption	Time

Medication	Dosage	Time

Activities ....

....

....

....

Caregiver Log Book

DATE ___/___/___   MON TUE WED THU FRI SAT SUN

Patient Name: ....

Caregiver: ....

Weight	Blood Pressure	Feeling

Food Consumption		Time

Medication	Dosage	Time

Activities

....

....

....

Caregiver Log Book

DATE _____ / ____ / _____   MON TUE WED THU FRI SAT SUN

Patient Name: ....

Caregiver: ....

Weight	Blood Pressure	Feeling

Food Consumption	Time

Medication	Dosage	Time

Activities

....

....

....

Caregiver Log Book

DATE ____/____/____   MON   TUE   WED   THU   FRI   SAT   SUN

Patient Name: ....

Caregiver: ....

Weight	Blood Pressure	Feeling

Food Consumption	Time

Medication	Dosage	Time

Activities

....

....

....

www.ingramcontent.com/pod-product-compliance
Lightning Source LLC
Chambersburg PA
CBHW051757200326
41597CB00025B/4593